OPIOID USE DISORDERS:

THERAPEUTIC MANUALS FOR HEALING AND RECUPERATION

Noogul Digital Publishing

Table of Contents

ABUSE, MISUSE AND ADDICTION OF OPIOID SUBSTANCES

Introduction

Drug misuse is a multifaceted problem that impacts individuals, families, and society as a whole. The physical, psychological, and social levels of individuals and society are all affected as a result of teenage drug addiction. Withdrawal symptoms include psychomotor, palpitation, perspiration, sleeplessness, restlessness, transitory hallucination or illusion, frustration, bodily and psychological ailments, and so on.

Drug misuse, cultivation, and trafficking of illicit narcotics and psychoactive substances are without a doubt a thorn in the flesh globally; it is a heinous deed in our society that causes confusion among the majority of our youth. It is a rapidly developing global issue that is currently a public health concern. Drug misuse poses a serious threat to the social, health, and economic fabric of families, societies, and even countries. Almost every country in the world is afflicted by citizens abusing one or more drugs.

Addiction, drug abuse, and misuse are all major public health issues. Many individuals frequently use these phrases interchangeably since they all relate to the use of illicit drugs as well as the improper use of legal substances (such as cigarettes, alcohol, and prescription medications). But each issue's interventions differ substantially from one another. The importance of accurately diagnosing a person's drug use is due to this. Medication on prescription has a lot of positive impacts. They can make us live longer, healthier lives when used properly under medical care. However, these same drugs have the capacity to have fatal results and serious adverse effects, particularly when overused or abused. Prescription drugs should only be taken by the individual for whom they are designed and exactly as directed due to this risk of damage.

Drug Misuse

Prescription medications are commonly related with drug misuse. Prescription medications are intended to be taken exactly as prescribed by doctors. This is because these medications might have negative side effects if the instructions are not followed.

Drug Misuse occurs when these drugs are used for purposes that are not in accordance with legal or medical norms.

- Taking the wrong dose
- Taking the medication at the wrong time
- Forgetting to take a dose
- Stopping the usage of a drug too soon
- Taking a medicine for reasons other than those indicated
- Taking a drug that was not prescribed to you

The FDA (2019) defines prescription medication MISUSE as failing to follow medical directions, although the individual using the medicine is not intending to "get high." If a person is unable to fall asleep after taking a single sleeping tablet, they may take another pill an hour later, reasoning, "That will do the job." Alternatively, a person may offer his headache medicine to a buddy in agony. Those are examples of drug abuse because, according to the FDA, the individual is treating oneself but not in accordance with the recommendations of their health care professionals. Prescription medication abuse can include: taking the wrong dose; taking a dose at the wrong time; forgetting to take a dose; and discontinuing medicine too soon, according to the Institute for Safe Medication Practices.

Drug Abuse

Drug abuse occurs when any psychoactive substance, including alcohol, illegal narcotics, and prescription medications, is used improperly to get high or hurt oneself. Since drug users exhibit profoundly changed thinking, behavior, and bodily functioning, it is also known as substance use disorder (SUD). According to the National Institute on Drug Abuse (NIDA, 2019), prescription drug abuse is the use of a medicine without a prescription, in a manner other than as directed, or for the experience or sensations it produces. For instance, drug abuse occurs when someone consumes a prescription medication in larger dosages than recommended in order to "get high" or have a pleasant or euphoric feeling.

The primary distinction between someone who misuses drugs and someone who abuses drugs is their purpose. The former consumes a medicine to cure a specific condition, whereas the latter consumes a substance to provoke specific emotions.

When a person fails to fall asleep after taking one sleeping pill and takes another one an hour later in the hopes that "it'll do the job," this is an example of drug abuse. But when someone uses sleeping drugs to regulate their moods, get a "high," or, in the worst-case circumstances, to attempt suicide, that is drug addiction.

Drug Addiction

Drug addiction, often referred to as severe SUD, is a brain illness that shows itself as the inability to stop using a substance despite the negative effects. Because they experience severe or incapacitating withdrawal symptoms when they stop using a substance, those who are addicted to drugs have a physical and/or psychological desire to use that substance.

Your brain and behavior are both impacted by the condition of addiction. Substance addiction makes it unable to resist the impulse to use the drug, regardless of how harmful it may be. The sooner you receive treatment for drug addiction, the better your chances are of avoiding some of the disease's more serious side effects.

Not simply heroin, cocaine, or other illicit narcotics are involved in drug addiction. Alcohol, nicotine, sleep aids, anti-anxiety drugs, and other legal substances can all cause addiction.

Drug misuse can take the form of addiction. The ability of the user to manage oneself is what distinguishes the two disorders. A person abusing drugs doesn't face a significant upheaval in their life since they still have control over it.

The majority, if not all, parts of a person's life are affected by an addiction, in contrast. Due to their substance use, they frequently skip job or school, put their families in financial or physical risk, experience health difficulties, encounter legal challenges, and engage in other hazardous behaviors. However, despite these, they are unable to alter their routines in order to improve their circumstances. This explains why a lot of drug addicts lose their jobs, end up homeless, or split up from their families. Some people's drug addiction even results in death.

Opioids

Opioids, sometimes known as narcotics, are pain relievers recommended by doctors to manage chronic or severe pain. People with persistent headaches and backaches, patients recuperating from surgery or enduring severe pain linked with cancer, and adults and children who have been gravely wounded in falls, traffic accidents, or other tragedies can all benefit from them.

Opioids are any natural or synthetic medications originating from or linked to the opium poppy, as well as any substance that works on opioid receptors in the brain. Opiates are a kind of opioid that is generated naturally from the opium poppy plant rather than synthetically.

Opioid medicines are designed to relieve pain, but they've been widely promoted and inappropriately administered, resulting in a slew of injuries and fatalities. Tramadol usage for a long time has been linked to liver and renal damage. High dosages of tramadol, in particular, can induce liver failure. Tramadol addiction, like other types of addiction, can result in severe behavioral changes as a result of obsessive drug seeking and obsession with taking the substance. Abuse of opioids can cause vomiting, mood swings, a loss of capacity to reason (cognitive function), and potentially respiratory failure, coma, or death. Opioids have a significant potential for addiction, and overdoses and deaths are prevalent

The opioid receptor system

Opioids attach to opioid receptors in the central nervous system, slowing the transmission of information between the brain and the body. Breathing and heart rate both slow down as a result of this. Dopamine is released as a result of opioid receptor stimulation, resulting in pleasure and pain alleviation.

A person's respiration and heart rate may drop to the point where they cease breathing, resulting in an overdose. Overdosing on opioids can result in death and serious damage, although it can be treated with CPR and naloxone.

Naloxone attaches to opioid receptors in the same way as other opioids do, but it has the opposite effect. It acts to counteract an overdose by preventing opioid receptors from binding to additional opioids (Growing et'al, 2014).

How are they used?
Opioids can be taken in a variety of ways; most opioid-based drugs are taken as tablets and are ingested. Orally, opioid-substitution therapy is available in liquid, pill, and film forms. Under the tongue, film forms disintegrate. Heroin is commonly injected, however it may also be smoked or snorted.

Many opioids are administered as pills, however they can also be administered as lozenges or lollipops. Others can be given by a vein, an injection, or an IV, while others can be given through a patch on the skin or a suppository (Growing et'al, 2014)..

How do opioids work?

Opioids bind to proteins on nerve cells in the brain, spinal cord, stomach, and other regions of the body called opioid receptors. When this happens, opioids block pain signals passed from the body to the brain via the spinal cord. Opioids have some hazards and can be extremely addicted, despite the fact that they can successfully treat pain. When opioids are used to treat chronic pain over a long period of time, the risk of addiction is very significant (Marshman er'al, 1998).

Opioid-based medications

Codeine (Panadeine®, Panadeine Forte®, and Nurofen Plus®), fentanyl, morphine, oxycodone (Endone® or OxyContin®), buprenorphine (Subutex® or Suboxone®), methadone, and tramadol are all examples of opioid-based drugs.

They produce the same pain-relieving effects as other opioids like heroin. Doctors often prescribe opioid-based drugs, and until 2018, certain lower-strength opioids could be purchased over the counter. Opioid-based drugs, on the other hand, are now only available with a prescription.

Many people are unaware that many pain-relieving drugs can lead to addiction. They can also induce overdose if they are misused or coupled with other central nervous system depressants like alcohol or benzodiazepines. In Australia, pharmaceutical opioids now account for more drug-related fatalities than any other medication class (Growing et'al, 2014)..

Effects of opioids

There is no such thing as a safe amount of drug consumption. Any medicine has a risk associated with it. When using any kind of medication, it's critical to be cautious.

Opioids affect people differently depending on their size, weight, and health; if they are habituated to taking them; whether they are taking other medicines at the same time; the amount taken; and the drug's potency.

People who take opioids may suffer the following symptoms:

- Complete relaxation
- Tiredness and clumsiness
- Befuddlement, slurred speech, sluggish breathing and heartbeat

If a excessive quantity is taken, the following symptoms may occur:

- Chilly, clammy skin
- Sluggish breathing
- Blue lips and fingertips
- Falling asleep ('nodding off')
- Death as a result of respiratory depression (Kleber, 2007).

Long-term effects include

- Harm to key organs such as the lungs, brain, and heart
- Greater tolerance
- Constipation
- Dependency

Using opioids with other drugs

The interactions between opioids and other medicines, whether over-the-counter or prescribed, can be unexpected and deadly, resulting in:

Opioids combined with alcohol, cannabis, or benzodiazepines cause slowed respiration and reduced brain activity, as well as an increased risk of overdosing.

Opioids combined with ice, speed, or ecstasy put the heart and kidneys under a lot of stress, and there's a higher chance of overdosing.

Health and safety

Use of opioids is likely to be more dangerous when:

- When opioids are used in combination with alcohol or other medications, particularly benzodiazepines or other opioids, they can impede respiration and raise the risk of overdose.
- A person is alone
- A person is driving or operating machinery, as a person's ability to gauge distance and space is highly restricted (in case medical assistance is required).
- The injection equipment is not sterile, thus an unaffected person should be present in case help is needed.

If you or someone you know is addicted to opioids, speak with your doctor about getting naloxone, the medicine that reverses opioid overdoses. In the event of an overdose, your friends or family members can be educated in overdose reversal (Growing et'al, 2014)..

Pain management strategies

Ask your doctor about a "pain management plan" and alternative non-medicine (like physical therapy) and non-opioid techniques (like paracetamol) you may employ to supplement your treatment and lessen your dependency on opioid-based drugs if you've been prescribed opioid-based meds.

Tolerance and dependence

Many medicines can lead to addiction if used over an extended period of time. Regular users of a substance might develop dependency and tolerance to it. This implies they'll have to take more of the medicine to have the same impact.

A drug's dependence might be psychological, physical, or both. When a person becomes addicted to a substance, it becomes significantly more essential than other things in their life. They are addicted to the substance and have a tough time quitting.

When people who are psychologically dependent on a substance are in certain situations, such as socializing with friends, they may feel compelled to use it.

When a person's body adapts to a substance and becomes accustomed to operating with the drug present, physical dependency develops (Kleber, 2007).

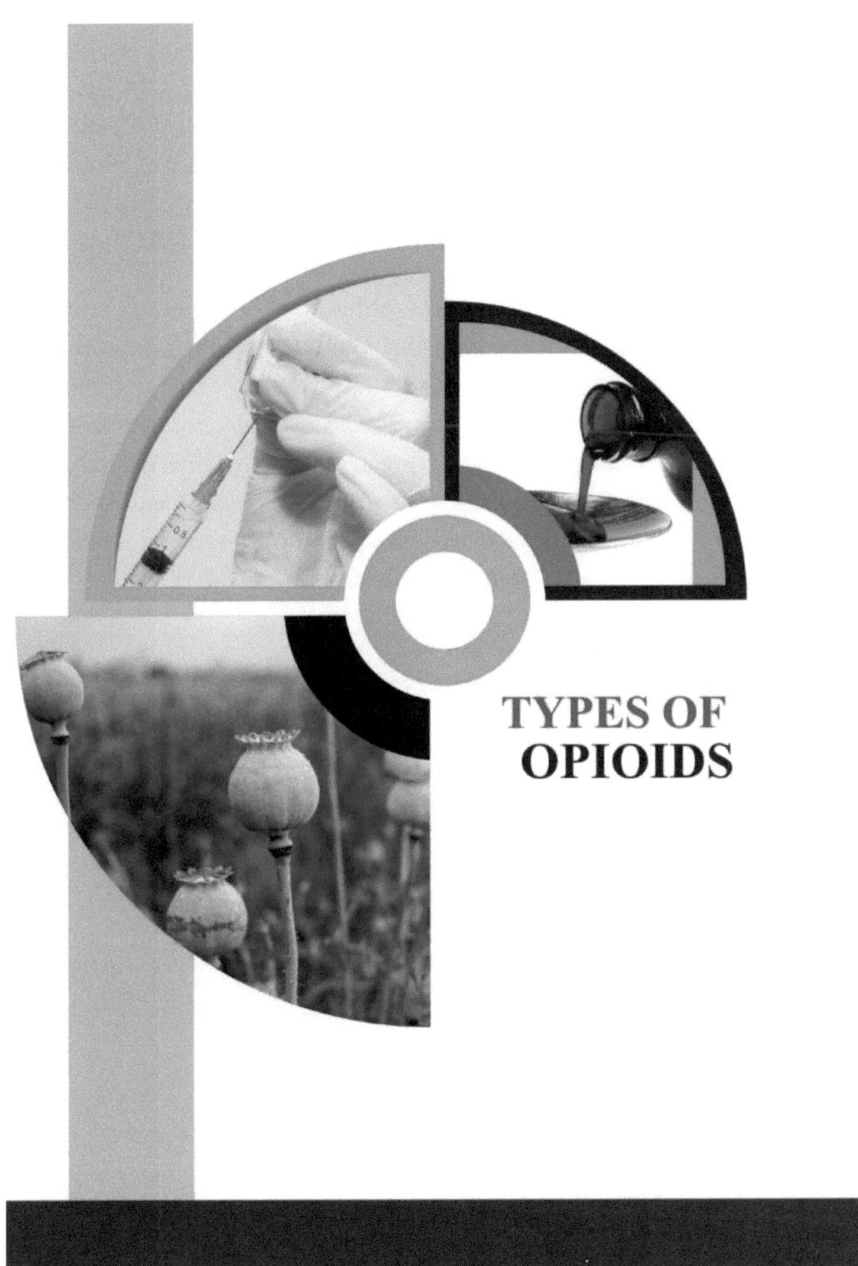

TYPES OF OPIOIDS

1.   BUPRENORPHINE

Buprenorphine (pronounced 'bew-pre-nor-feen') is a prescription medication used to treat opioid addiction. It's used as a substitute in the treatment of heroin and methadone addiction. The Food and Drug Administration (FDA) has authorized buprenorphine as a medication-assisted therapy for opioid use disorder (OUD) (MAT).

Buprenorphine, like other drugs, should be provided as part of a comprehensive treatment plan that includes counseling and other behavioral treatments to ensure that patients receive a holistic therapy. Pharmacotherapy is the process of replacing a prescription medicine to treat a drug addiction in this way. Pharmacotherapy helps to stabilize the lives of persons who are addicted on heroin and other opioids, as well as lessen the consequences associated with drug use, by avoiding physical withdrawal (Growing et'al, 2014).

Chemical Structure of Buprenorphine

Buprenorphine medication can be used to:

- Aid withdrawal from heroin and methadone;
- Lessen the urge for heroin (buprenorphine maintenance); and
- Manage severe pain.

Buprenorphine is the first OUD medicine that may be prescribed or delivered in a doctor's office, greatly expanding treatment options.

After completing specialized training, qualified practitioners can dispense or prescribe buprenorphine for the treatment of opioid use disorders (OUD) in settings other than opioid treatment programs (OTP) under the Drug Addiction Treatment Act of 2000 (DATA 2000), the Comprehensive Addiction and Recovery Act (CARA), and the Substance Use-Disorder Prevention Opioid Recovery and Treatment for Patients and Communities (SUPPORT) Act.

Other names

Pharmaceutical name

There are four formulations of buprenorphine available for people on pharmacotherapy treatment:

- Suboxone Sublingual Film® – A combination of buprenorphine and naloxone (also known as Narcan®). This is the most widely used form.
- Subutex Sublingual Tablets® – Contains only buprenorphine.
- Buvidal® is a modified release formulation of buprenorphine for administration by subcutaneous (SC) injection once a week (Buvidal® Weekly) or once a month (Buvidal® Monthly).
- Sublocade® is an extended-release formulation of BPN, administered monthly by Subcutaneous injection (Under the Skin) (Lintzeris et'al, 2019).

Slang names

Bup, B, subs, bupe, orange

How is it used?

Suboxone Sublingual Film® is a rectangular, orange film with a lime flavor that is put under the tongue to dissolve. If the film is eaten or ingested, it will not function correctly.

Subutex Sublingual Tablets® are also put beneath the tongue to dissolve, and if chewed or swallowed, they will not operate effectively.

How effective is it?

Treatment with buprenorphine is more likely to be effective if it is part of a larger treatment plan that addresses the body, mind, and environment in which opioids were used.

Treatment could involve buprenorphine, counseling, alternative treatments, and the formation of a positive support network of colleagues, friends, and a support group, for example.

Buprenorphine maintenance Therapy

Buprenorphine maintenance therapy (BMT) is a medication-assisted treatment for those who are addicted to opioids. The aims of BMT are to reduce the risk of overdose from illegal opioid use by alleviating withdrawal symptoms, suppressing opiate effects and cravings, and decreasing the danger of overdose.

Because buprenorphine maintenance may not be right for everyone, it's crucial to consult with a doctor or a drug counselor to determine the best course of action (SAMHSA 2019)..

Therapy Component

Opioids, such as heroin or morphine, cause the body to release too much dopamine. Because opiates are required to keep the opioid receptor in the brain occupied, users grow addicted to the substance. Buprenorphine, like methadone, acts by occupying this receptor and inhibiting the euphoria associated with illegal opioid drug usage. Because methadone is a complete agonist, it has a higher agonist action at opioid receptor sites, whereas buprenorphine is a partial agonist and has a lesser agonist effect (Lintzeris et'al, 2019)..

Because it is a partial agonist, buprenorphine has a lesser agonist activity at opioid receptor sites. Buprenorphine's effects rise when the drug's dosage is raised, until the effects approach a plateau at moderate levels and no longer expand (known as the ceiling effect). Buprenorphine's maximum effects are generally achieved at doses of 16–32 milligrams (mg). Because methadone is a complete agonist, it has a greater agonist impact. However, there is no limit to how much methadone may make you feel, which can lead to lethal overdoses if you use it illegally.

It has a lesser risk of addiction, overdose, and adverse effects than full opioid agonists, buprenorphine can be utilized as a viable pharmaceutical alternative to methadone. The dosage schedule is another advantage. Buprenorphine's effects are not as powerful as methadone's, but they stay longer. While methadone must be taken every day, buprenorphine can be given every two days. This can be beneficial in BMT because patients who are addicted to opioids may be put off by therapy that needs daily medication and clinic visits, whereas buprenorphine allows for alternate day administration.

Buprenorphine's effects rise when the drug's dosage is raised; however, at moderate levels, the effects plateau and do not continue to expand (known as the ceiling effect). Illicit drug usage can result in lethal overdoses since methadone has no upper limit on the degree of effects it can produce. Because it has a lesser risk of addiction, overdose, and adverse effects than full opioid agonists, buprenorphine can be utilized as a viable pharmaceutical alternative to methadone.

BMT is divided into three stages: *induction, stabilization, and maintenance.* Patients are medically supervised during the induction period while they begin buprenorphine medication. After individuals have significantly reduced or quit abusing opioids, the stability phase starts. They no longer have cravings and have minimal, if any, adverse symptoms throughout this time. During this time, the dose may be changed. Once patients have reached a stable dosage of buprenorphine, the maintenance phase starts. The amount of time that patients get BMT varies from person to person and may be endless (SAMHSA 2019).

BMT can also involve extensive rehabilitation services such as group therapy, individual counseling, medical services, and referrals to community-based agencies, in addition to medicine.

Advantages of buprenorphine maintenance over heroin use

Buprenorphine has a limited risk for misuse and is widely available for usage in offices. The high expense and potential lack of efficacy in individuals who require large methadone dosages are also disadvantages.

- Buprenorphine is unlikely to cause an overdose when used alone.
- Buprenorphine maintenance allows a person to remain stable while making beneficial life adjustments.

- Health concerns, particularly those associated to injecting, such as HIV, hepatitis B and C viruses, skin infections, and vein difficulties, are decreased or prevented.
- Because buprenorphine's effects are long-lasting, doses are only needed once a day, sometimes even less often.
- Buprenorphine is a lot less expensive than heroin .

Effects of buprenorphine

Constipation, dizziness, sleepiness, headache, and nausea are all common buprenorphine adverse effects. Drug withdrawal, lethargy, vomiting, hyperhidrosis, and xerostomia are some of the other negative effects.

There is no such thing as a safe amount of drug consumption. Any medicine has a risk associated with it. Even drugs can have unintended consequences. When using any kind of medication, it's critical to be cautious.

Buprenorphine affects people differently depending on their size, weight, and health, as well as if they are habituated to taking it and whether they are taking other medicines at the same time (SAMHSA 2019).

Side effects

The following are the most prevalent buprenorphine adverse effects:

- Lack of appetite, nausea, and vomiting
- Stomach discomfort
- Skin rashes, itching, or hives
- Teeth decay
- Changes in periods (menstruation)

-   Reduced sex desire (males and females)
-   Weight gain (particularly for females).

Withdrawal

Withdrawal from long-term buprenorphine usage can cause symptoms that are comparable to those of heroin withdrawal. To avoid discomfort and unpleasant side effects, it is suggested that buprenorphine withdrawal be done gradually under medical supervision. The following are examples of withdrawal symptoms that differ from person to person:

-   cold or flu-like symptoms
-   headaches
-   sweating
-   aches and pains
-   inability to sleep
-   nausea
-   mood fluctuations and
-   loss of appetite

The first 2 to 5 days are generally the most intense. Some modest side effects might continue for weeks (SAMHSA 2019).

2. CODEINE

Codeine, like morphine and hydrocodone, is a narcotic pain reliever and cough suppressant. Furthermore, throughout the body, a little quantity of codeine gets converted to morphine. Codeine's exact mechanism of action is unknown; however, like morphine, it attaches to opioid receptors in the brain, which are vital for relaying pain sensations throughout the body and brain. Although codeine improves pain tolerance and reduces discomfort, the patient nevertheless feels pain. Codeine reduces pain while simultaneously causing sleepiness, drowsiness, and respiratory depression. For more effective pain management, codeine is commonly coupled with acetaminophen (Tylenol) or aspirin. Codeine was cleared by the FDA in 1950 (Cairns et'al, 2019).

Chemical Structure of Codeine

Codeine has the potential to become addictive. Follow the instructions for taking codeine strictly. Do not take more of it, take it more frequently, or take it in any other way than your doctor has prescribed. Discuss your pain treatment objectives, length of therapy, and other approaches to control your pain with your healthcare professional while taking codeine. Tell your doctor if you or anyone in your family consumes or has consumed significant quantities of alcohol, uses or has consumed street drugs, has misused prescription medications, has experienced an overdose, or has experienced depression or another mental disorder (Cairns et'al, 2019)..

Why is this medication prescribed?

Codeine is a pain reliever that is used to treat mild to severe pain. It's also used to treat coughing, generally in conjunction with other drugs. Codeine can aid with symptom relief, but it will not address the underlying cause of the symptoms or hasten recovery. Codeine belongs to the opiate (narcotic) analgesics and antitussives classes of drugs. When codeine is used to alleviate pain, it alters the way the brain and nervous system react to the sensation. When codeine is used to treat coughing, it works by reducing activity in the brain area that produces coughing.

Codeine is also included in cough and cold treatments in conjunction with acetaminophen (Capital and Codeine, Tylenol with Codeine), aspirin, carisoprodol, and promethazine. If you're taking a codeine combination medicine, read the label carefully to learn about all of the components and contact your doctor or pharmacist for further information (Mental Health and drug and Alcohol Office, 2018).

Mode of Administration of Codeine

Codeine is usually swallowed and comes in different forms, including:

- Tablets
- Capsules
- Suppositories

- soluble powders and tablets
- liquids.

Other names

Codeine may also be known by a brand or trade name. Some common examples are:

Generic name	Brand names
Aspirin and codeine	Aspalgin®, Codral Cold & Flu Original®
Ibuprofen and codeine	Nurofen Plus®
Paracetamol and codeine	Panadeine Forte®, Panamax Co®
Paracetamol, codeine and doxylamine	Mersyndol® and Mersyndol Forte®, Panalgesic®

Effects of codeine

Codeine is available as a tablet, a pill, and a solution (liquid) to take by mouth (alone or in combination with other drugs). It's commonly taken every 4 to 6 hours, depending on the situation. Follow the directions on your prescription label carefully, and if there is anything you don't understand, ask your doctor or pharmacist to explain it to you.

There is no such thing as a safe amount of drug consumption. Any substance has the potential to have undesired side effects, and drugs are no exception. When using any kind of medication, it's critical to be cautious.

Codeine affects people differently depending on their size, weight, and health; if they are habituated to taking it; whether they are taking other medications at the same time; and the amount consumed (Van et'al, 2017).

Negative effects

The following are the most common codeine side effects:

- Dizziness
- Tiredness
- Confusion, Difficulty Concentrating
- Euphoria
- Restlessness
- Blurred vision
- Dry mouth
- Limbs feeling heavy or stiff
- Sweating
- Mild allergic rash, itching and hives
- Low blood pressure
- Decreased heart rate, palpitations
- Stomach-ache, nausea, vomiting, constipation
- Difficulty urinating

With sustained therapy, these adverse effects may fade. However, if they continue, you should seek medical advice.

Overdose

Taking some drugs while receiving codeine therapy may raise your chance of developing breathing issues or other serious, life-threatening respiratory problems, as well as drowsiness or coma. If you are taking or intend to take any of the following drugs, tell your doctor:

- benzodiazepines such alprazolam (Xanax),
- diazepam (Diastat, Valium),
- estazolam,
- flurazepam,
- lorazepam (Ativan), and
- triazolam (Halcion);
- carbamazepine (Carbatrol, Epitol, Equetro, Tegretol, Teril);

Some antifungal medications like

- ketoconazole; erythromycin (Erytab, Erythrocin);

Your doctor may need to adjust your medication levels and will keep a close eye on you. If you take codeine with any of these drugs and have unusual dizziness, lightheadedness, excessive drowsiness, delayed or difficult breathing, or unresponsiveness, call your doctor or seek emergency medical help right away. If you are unable to seek treatment on your own, make sure your caregiver or family members arc aware of which symptoms may be dangerous so they can contact a doctor or seek emergency medical help.

If you drink alcohol or use illicit drugs while receiving codeine therapy, you're more likely to develop these serious, life-threatening adverse effects. During your therapy, avoid drinking alcohol, using alcohol-containing prescription or nonprescription medicines, or using illegal narcotics. If you are pregnant or intend to become pregnant, tell your doctor. If you consume codeine on a regular basis while pregnant, your baby may have life-threatening withdrawal symptoms after birth.

Do not give your medicine to anybody else. Other individuals who take your prescription, especially youngsters, may be harmed or killed by codeine (Van et'al, 2017).

You may overdose if your codeine dose is too high. If you or someone you know is experiencing any of the following symptoms, call an ambulance right away (ambulance officers do not need to engage the police):

- Difficulty to pass urine
- Severe constipation and bowel obstruction
- Agitation
- Cold, clammy skin with a blue tint
- Mental numbness
- Extremely slow, shallow breathing
- Hallucinations and occasionally convulsions
- Coma and death

Long-term effects of codeine

Regular use of codeine may eventually cause:

- Constipation
- Decreased sex desire
- Irregular periods
- Tension and muscle spasms
- Needing more to get the same effect
- Tolerance and dependency on codeine
- Financial, job, and social issues

The interactions between codeine and other substances, such as alcohol, prescription pharmaceuticals, and over-the-counter medications, are frequently unexpected.

When codeine is used with alcohol, it might produce mental fogginess, slowed breathing, and decreased coordination (Van et'al, 2017)..

Withdrawal

Giving off codeine after a lengthy period of use is difficult since the body must adjust to life without it. Please seek medical advice if you have any concerns.

Codeine is addicting (addictive). When used for short-term pain treatment, mental and physical reliance are possible but improbable. If codeine is used during pregnancy, the infant may have opioid withdrawal syndrome, which can be fatal if not addressed.

Withdrawal symptoms may appear if codeine is suddenly stopped after a lengthy period of usage. To avoid withdrawal symptoms, the dose of codeine should be progressively tapered.

Withdrawal symptoms often begin a few hours after the last dosage and peak between 48 and 72 hours.

- Dilated pupils
- Abdominal cramps, diarrhoea, nausea, vomiting •
- Lack of appetite
- Flu-like symptoms such as runny nose, sneezing, sweating, chills, and fever

- Yawning and difficulty sleeping
- Trembling, aching muscles and joints
- Goosebumps
- Restlessness, irritability, nervousness, depression (Cairns et'al, 2019)

3. BUPRENORPHINE - LONG ACTING INJECTABLE

Buprenorphine is a kind of opioid that is used to treat opioid addiction, acute pain, and chronic pain. It can be injected (intravenous and subcutaneous), used as a skin patch (transdermal), or implanted under the tongue (sublingual), in the cheek (buccal), via injection (intravenous and subcutaneous), as a skin patch (transdermal), or as an implant.

In the treatment of heroin and methadone addiction, buprenorphine is used as a substitute. Pharmacotherapy is the process of replacing a prescription medicine to treat a drug addiction in this way. Pharmacotherapy helps to stabilize the lives of persons who are addicted on heroin and other opioids, as well as lessen the consequences associated with drug use, by avoiding physical withdrawal.

The Food and Drug Administration (FDA) has authorized buprenorphine as a Medication-Assisted Therapy (MAT) for opioid use disorder (OUD). Buprenorphine, like all other MAT drugs, should be provided as part of a complete treatment plan that also includes counseling and other behavioral treatments to give patients a holistic approach (SAMHSA, 2019).

Opioid dependency is treated with buprenorphine and a combination of buprenorphine and naloxone (addiction to opioid drugs, including heroin and narcotic painkillers). This medication has proved effective in treating OUD and may be prescribed or delivered in a doctor's office, greatly expanding treatment options.

Buprenorphine belongs to the opioid partial agonist-antagonist class of drugs, while naloxone belongs to the opioid antagonist class. When someone quits taking opioid medicines, buprenorphine alone or in combination with naloxone works to reduce withdrawal symptoms by having similar effects to the drugs (SAMHSA, 2019)..

What is depot buprenorphine?

Depot buprenorphine is a novel long-acting version of buprenorphine, an established opioid medication. Buvidal® and Sublocade®, two types of Long-Acting Injectable Buprenorphine, become available in April 2020. They are delivered as subcutaneous (under the skin) injections that progressively release buprenorphine into the body and are available in weekly or monthly dosages (Growing et'al, 2014).

It is injected as a liquid by a treatment provider or health expert, and once within the body, it transforms into a solid gel known as a depot (dee-poh).

Other names

Pharmaceutical names

Buvidal®, Sublocade®

Slang names

Bup, B, subs, bupe, orange

How is it used?

Buprenorphine is available in the form of a sublingual tablet. The buprenorphine and naloxone combination is available as a sublingual tablet (Zubsolv), a sublingual film (Suboxone), and a buccal film (Bunavail) to place between the gum and cheek. These products are normally used once a day after your doctor sets an acceptable dose. Take or apply buprenorphine or buprenorphine plus naloxone at the same time every day to make it easier to remember. Follow the directions on your prescription label carefully, and if there is anything you don't understand, ask your doctor or pharmacist to explain it to you. Take buprenorphine, buprenorphine plus naloxone, or buprenorphine and naloxone precisely as prescribed.

Buvidal® Weekly/Monthly

Buvidal® is a prolonged-release subcutaneous injection containing buprenorphine. It is available in two different formulations which are administered at either weekly (8 mg, 16 mg, 24 mg, 32 mg) or monthly (64 mg, 96 mg, 128 mg, 160 mg) intervals. The weekly and monthly Buvidal® products are differentiated by the colour of the cardboard boxes, and the text "once weekly" or "once monthly" printed on the respective boxes (NIHCE, 2019).

A healthcare practitioner administers Buvidal Weekly and Monthly injections in a hospital, clinic, or drugstore. Only a doctor's prescription is required to obtain this medication.

You must be stable on sublingual (under the tongue) buprenorphine or buprenorphine/naloxone for at least seven days before starting Buvidal Weekly or Monthly.

The day after your final dosage of sublingual therapy, you can begin taking Buvidal Weekly or Monthly.

Buvidal Weekly or Monthly will be prescribed to you by your doctor or health care provider at the appropriate starting dose.

Depending on your requirements, your doctor may reduce or increase the dose throughout therapy. During the dosage term, you can obtain more Buvidal Weekly doses if needed.

How it will be given

Buvidal is injected beneath the skin (subcutaneously) in the buttock, thigh, belly, or upper arm on a weekly or monthly basis.

Sublocade®

SUBLOCADE® (buprenorphine extended-release) injection for subcutaneous use (CIII) is a prescription medicine for adults with moderate to severe addiction (dependence) to opioid drugs (prescription or illegal) who have received an oral transmucosal (under the tongue or inside the cheek) buprenorphine-containing medicine at a dose that controls withdrawal symptoms for at least 7 days. SUBLOCADE should be used as part of a comprehensive treatment strategy that includes counseling.

SUBLOCADE can cause significant and life-threatening respiratory issues, especially if you also take or use other medications or substances. SUBLOCADE may lead to significant and perhaps fatal respiratory issues. If you're having a medical emergency, call the hospital straight immediately if you feel: .

You're dizzy and faint, and you're perplexed.

Feeling drowsy or clumsy, with hazy vision and slurred speech, and breathing more slowly than usual

Can't think clearly or well (NIHCE, 2019).

How effective is it?

If Buvidal or Sublocade is administered as part of a complete treatment program that treats the body, mind, and environment in which opioids were used, it is more likely to be successful.

Treatment could involve buprenorphine, counseling, alternative treatments, and the formation of a positive support network of colleagues, friends, and a support group, for example.

Advantages of buprenorphine maintenance over heroin use

Buprenorphine is a partial opioid agonist. At low to moderate dosages, it causes feelings of euphoria or respiratory depression. These effects are milder with buprenorphine than with complete opioid agonists like methadone and heroin.

Buprenorphine is both safe and effective when used as directed. Buprenorphine has unique pharmacological features that serve to Reduce the symptoms of physical opioid dependency, such as withdrawal symptoms and cravings; Increased safety in overdose situations and Reduced risk of abuse.

Buprenorphine is unlikely to cause an overdose if used alone. Maintenance on buprenorphine allows a person to remain stable while making constructive adjustments in their lives. Health concerns, particularly those connected to injecting, such as HIV, hepatitis B and C viruses, skin infections, and vein difficulties, are decreased or prevented.

Because the effects are long-lasting, just weekly or monthly doses are necessary. Buprenorphine is a lot less expensive than heroin.

Effects of buprenorphine

Because buprenorphine is a synthetic opioid that gives the euphoric effects desired by opiate addicts, it may be abused in both of the authorized forms for treating opiate addiction. While buprenorphine can be overdosed, it is safer than methadone due to its ceiling effect and lower degree of respiratory depression. Buprenorphine is also more difficult to divert than methadone due to the multiple protections in place. Methadone misuse, whether diverted or legally prescribed, is becoming a major danger, as indicated by the rising fatality rates connected with it.

When buprenorphine and heroin are combined, the effects of both drugs are amplified, but when buprenorphine and methadone are combined, the effects of both drugs are amplified. As a result, individuals who are presently on methadone for opiate addiction treatment may find diverted buprenorphine appealing .

The product's qualities for sustained release should be taken into account while starting and finishing a treatment. Patients with concurrent medications and/or comorbidities should be closely watched for any indications or symptoms of toxicity, overdose, or withdrawal brought on by changing buprenorphine levels (Health Improvement Scotland, 2022).

Buprenorphine affects everyone differently, based on:

- size, weight and health
- whether the person is used to taking it
- whether other drugs are taken around the same time
- the amount taken.

Side effects

The following are some of the most prevalent negative effects associated with buprenorphine use:

- Flu-like symptoms such as chills, fever, sore throat, coughing, runny nose, and sweating
- Unsettled stomach and diarrhoea
- Responses at the injection site (redness, discomfort, itching, nodule just beneath the skin)
- Abnormal liver function
- Respiratory depression
- Central nervous system (CNS) depression
- Dependence
- Serotonin syndrome
- Hepatitis and hepatic events
- Drug withdrawal syndrome
- Precipitation of opioid withdrawal syndrome
- Hepatic impairment

- Renal impairment
- QT prolongation

Class effects of opioids. (Health Improvement Scotland, 2022)

Buprenorphine has a number of serious adverse effects, including:

- Distress in the lungs
- Overdose
- Insufficiency of the adrenal glands
- Dependence
- Withdrawal
- Itching, discomfort, swelling, and nerve damage are all symptoms of nerve injury (implant)
- Injection site discomfort (injection)
- Neonatal abstinence syndrome (NAS) is a condition in which a baby is born (in newborns)

Other less common side effects include:

- Dental problems
- Headache, migraine
- Sleepiness, dizziness, fainting, vertigo
- Abnormal vision
- Difficulty sleeping
- Chest Pain
- Pain in joints, muscles, back, stomach
- Cramps
- Flushing, feeling warm
- Difficulty breathing
- Cough, respiratory infection

- Nausea, vomiting, constipation
- Diarrhoea, poor appetite
- Rash and itching
- Low sex drive, impotence

If you notice any of the aforementioned adverse effects, or any additional negative effects, you should contact your doctor right once.

4.   FENTANYL

Fentanyl is a 50-100 times stronger synthetic opioid than morphine. Fentanyl was created as a pain reliever for cancer patients, and it was administered to the skin as a patch. Fentanyl is also diverted for misuse due to its potent opioid effects. Fentanyl is added to heroin to boost its strength, or be disguised as very strong heroin. Many users mistakenly assume they are buying heroin when they are actually buying fentanyl, which often leads to overdose fatalities. Mexico is the primary source of illegally made fentanyl (Darke et'al, 2019).

Chemical Structure of Fentanyl

Pharmaceutical fentanyl and illicitly made fentanyl are the two forms of fentanyl. Both of these substances are classified as synthetic opioids. Doctors use pharmaceutical fentanyl to alleviate extreme pain, particularly after surgery and in advanced-stage cancer.

However, the majority of recent fentanyl-related overdose incidents have been attributed to illicitly made fentanyl, which is sold on the black market for its heroin-like effects. Because of its extraordinary strength, it is frequently added to other drugs, making them cheaper, more potent, more addictive, and more hazardous (Darke et'al, 2019).

Illicitly manufactured fentanyl

On the drug market, Illicitly Manufactured Fentanyl (IMF) comes in a variety of forms, including liquid and powder.

Fentanyl powder resembles a variety of different medicines. It's sometimes combined with other substances like heroin, cocaine, and methamphetamine and packaged into tablets that look like prescription painkillers. Drugs laced with fentanyl are exceedingly hazardous, and many patients are unaware that their medications include fentanyl.

IMF can be available in nasal sprays, ocular drops, and drips on paper or little candies in liquid form.

Street Names

Apace, China Girl, China Town, China White, Dance Fever, Goodfellas, Great Bear, He-Man, Poison and Tango & Cash,

What it looks like

Fentanyl comes in a variety of forms. Fentanyl is a pharmaceutical that is used to treat acute and chronic pain. Illicit fentanyl can be produced for sale on the black market.

Medicinal use

Medicinal fentanyl comes in a number of different forms and strengths including:

- transdermal patches (Durogesic®, APO-fentanyl® and generic versions)
- lozenges/lollipops (Actiq®)
- intravenous injection (Sublimaze® B. BRAUN FENTANYL®).

Illicit use

Fentanyl is illegally used by certain people who take it from the patch and inject it. This is particularly dangerous since estimating dosage size is quite difficult.

Fentanyl can be 'diverted,' which means it is not used as indicated or provided or sold to a third party after being prescribed by a medical expert.

Prescription fentanyl can be 'diverted' if people:

- Receive medicine from another doctor without a prescription through their profession (e.g., healthcare professionals);
- Use their own prescribed medication recreationally;
- Utilize medication intended for someone else

To improve its strength, fentanyl is occasionally combined with other medications. Fentanyl produced illegally can be sold as a stand-alone product, a low-cost addition to improve the strength of other illicit substances like heroin, or as counterfeit pharmaceuticals (such as oxycodone®).

Effects of fentanyl

There is no such thing as a safe amount of drug consumption. Any medicine has a risk associated with it. When using any kind of medication, it's critical to be cautious.

Fentanyl provides symptoms such as relaxation, euphoria, pain alleviation, sedation, disorientation, sleepiness, dizziness, nausea and vomiting, urine retention, pupillary constriction, and respiratory depression, similar to other opioid analgesics (Darke et'al, 2019).

Fentanyl affects people differently depending on their size, weight, and health; if they are habituated to taking it; whether they are taking other medicines at the same time; the amount consumed; and the drug's potency (varies between drug form e.g. patches, lozenges or injection).

Its effects may include:

- Exhilaration
- Pain alleviation
- Nausea, vomiting
- Constipation and/or diarrhea
- Decreased appetite
- Wind, indigestion, cramps
- Sleepiness, confusion
- Weakness or exhaustion
- Dizziness
- Headache
- Unclear or slurred speech
- Impaired balance
- Sluggish pulse and/or blood pressure (inflammation, itch, swelling at patch site).

Fentanyl Overdose

The most frequent medications implicated in overdose deaths are fentanyl and other synthetic opioids. It can be fatal in even tiny dosages. Every day, approximately 150 individuals die from overdoses caused by synthetic opioids like fentanyl. (Hedegaard et'al, 2021)

Fentanyl levels in drugs may be lethal, and you wouldn't be able to see, taste, or smell it. Unless you test your medicines using fentanyl test strips, it's practically hard to detect if they've been laced with fentanyl.

Test strips are cheap and may provide results in as little as 5 minutes, which might be the difference between life and death. Even if the test comes back negative, be cautious since test strips may miss more powerful fentanyl-like compounds such as carfentanil. (Banta, 2021)

If you develop any of the following symptoms, call an ambulance right away:

- Chest discomfort
- Slower breathing
- Blue lips and complexion
- Seizure
- Passing Out
- Coma
- Death.

Naloxone (commonly known as Narcan®) reverses the effects of opiates in the event of an overdose (including fentanyl).

Naloxone is offered as a fast-acting nasal spray or a preloaded multiple dosage syringe and is accessible over the counter.

Health professionals, family or household members, and peers can all administer it. For further information, talk to your pharmacist or chemist.

There is an increased risk of:

- Tetanus while injecting medicines.
- Infection.
- Injury to the veins

If you share needles, you run the risk of contracting:

- hepatitis B.
- Hepatitis C (A kind of hepatitis that affects the liver).
- AIDS and HIV.

Long-term effects

Regular use of fentanyl may cause:

- Instability of mood
- Low libido
- Constipation
- Menstrual difficulties
- Respiratory problems (Hedegaard et'al, 2021)

Using fentanyl with other drugs

Fentanyl's interactions with other pharmaceuticals, including over-the-counter and prescription prescriptions, can be unexpected and deadly, and can result in:

- **Fentanyl with alcohol** intensifies the negative effects and raises the risk of respiratory depression.
- **Antidepressants including fentanyl and monoamine oxidase inhibitors (MAOI)** may cause severe and unexpected responses. MAOIs were the first antidepressants to be created,

although they have now been mostly supplanted by safer and less side-effect-prone alternatives.
- **Fentanyl with benzodiazepines** may increase sedation and respiratory difficulty.

Withdrawal

Giving off fentanyl after a lengthy period of usage is difficult since the body must adjust to life without it. Please seek medical advice if you have any concerns.

Withdrawal symptoms often begin 12 hours after the last dosage and persist approximately a week. The first three days will be the most difficult. Symptoms include:

- Goose flesh/bumps
- Chills alternating with flushing and excessive sweating
- Irritability
- Insomnia
- Loss of appetite
- Yawning and sneezing
- Watery eyes and runny nose
- Vomiting and nausea
- Diarrhea
- Increased heart rate and blood pressure
- Bone and muscle pains
- General weakness
- Depression (Banta, 2021)

5.   HEROIN

Pure heroin (diacetylmorphine), a white powder with a bitter flavor that is abused for its euphoric effects, is a white powder with a bitter taste. Heroin is generated from the morphine alkaloid found in the opium poppy plant (Papaver somniferum) and is about 2 to 3 times more powerful than morphine. Typically, it is injected, smoked, or snorted up the nose. It has euphoric (rush) effects, as well as anti-anxiety and pain-relieving characteristics (Black et'al, 2014).

Chemical Structure of Heroin

The majority of illegal heroin is marketed as a white or brownish powder that has been "cut" with other drugs or substances like sugar, starch, powdered milk, or quinine. Strychnine or other poisons can also be used to cut it. This is the shape into which the substance is injected.

Potent opioids like fentanyl and carfentanyl have been discovered cut into heroin sold on the streets, and they can be fatal to an unwitting user.

Heroin is available in a variety of forms, including:

- Fine white powder
- Granules that are gritty and off-white
- Teeny-tiny 'rock' bits in a light brown color.

It's commonly offered in 'caps' or grams (a little amount, usually enough for one injection). It's commonly packed in 'foils' (aluminum foil wrapping) or little, colorful balloons.

Another form is "black tar" it's sticky, similar to roofing tar, or hard, similar to coal. It can range in hue from dark brown to black. It's generally smoked or snorted in this form. Abusers are frequently at risk of overdosing or dying because they are unaware of the drug's true potency or ingredients (Black et'al, 2014).

Other names

Smack, gear, hammer, the dragon, H, dope, junk, harry, horse, black tar, white dynamite, homebake, china white, Chinese H, poison, Dr Harry

How is it used?

Heroin is normally injected into a vein, although it may also be smoked ('chasing the dragon,') or mixed with cigarettes and cannabis. The effects are normally noticed within seconds of injecting or smoking it, but if inhaled, it will take 10 to 15 minutes.

Effects of heroin

There is no such thing as a safe amount of drug consumption. Any medicine has a risk associated with it. When using any kind of medication, it's critical to be cautious.

Heroin affects people differently depending on their size, weight, and health; if they are habituated to taking it; whether they are taking other drugs at the same time; the amount consumed; and the potency of the substance (it varies from batch to batch).

The following are the primary effects of heroin, which generally last three to five hours:

-   Slurred and sluggish speech
-   Slow breathing and pulse
-   Dry lips
-   Small pupils
-   Poor appetite and vomiting
-   Diminished sex desire
-   Tremendous pleasure and pain alleviation
-   Relaxation, tiredness, and clumsiness
-   Befuddlement
-   Detached sensations

When you inject drugs, you're more likely to get: Tetanus, infection, and vein damage are all possibilities.

Sugar, starch, or powdered milk are common additions in heroin that can block blood arteries leading to the lungs, liver, kidneys, or brain, causing irreversible harm (Guerin, 2018).

When you share needles, you run the danger of:

-   Hepatitis B
-   Hepatitis C
-   HIV and AIDS

Heroin Overdose

You might overdose if you consume a huge amount of heroin or have a very potent batch.

If you or someone else is experiencing any of the symptoms described below, call an ambulance right away (ambulance personnel do not need to engage the police):

- Severe sleepiness or falling asleep ('going on the nod')
- Difficulty concentrating
- Tiny ('pinned') pupils
- A strong desire to urinate yet difficulty doing so
- Itchiness
- Blood pressure that is too low
- Unsteady heartbeat
- Hypothermia
- Fainting out
- Death
- Chilly, clammy skin
- Sluggish breathing, blue lips and fingertips

In the event of an overdose, naloxone (commonly known as Narcan®) reverses the effects of heroin and other opioids. Naloxone can be injected intramuscularly (directly into a muscle) or sprayed into the nose

Coming down

The following symptoms may occur in the days following heroin use:

- Irritability

- Depression.

Long-term effects

Regular heroin use can lead to:

- Intense sadness
- Irregular periods and difficulty having children
- No sex drive, erectile dysfunction, and infertility in men
- Constipation
- Dental issues
- Damaged heart, lungs, liver, and brain
- Vein damage and skin, heart, and lung infections from injecting
- Needing to use more to achieve the same effect
- Heroin dependence
- Financial, work, or social problems (Guerin, 2018).

Using heroin with other drugs

Taking heroin with other substances, such as over-the-counter or prescribed pharmaceuticals, can have unpredictable and severe consequences, including:

- **Heroin combined with ice, speed, or ecstasy** causes severe heart and kidney damage, as well as an increased chance of overdosing.
- **Heroin combined with alcohol, cannabis, or benzodiazepines** can cause respiration to become labored and finally cease. Aspiration of vomit is also a possibility (Black et'al, 2014).

Withdrawal

Heroin is a highly addictive substance. People who use heroin on a regular basis acquire a tolerance to the drug, requiring greater and/or more frequent dosages to achieve the desired effects. When long-term use of a drug creates problems, such as health problems and failure to perform duties at work, school, or family, it is called a substance use disorder (SUD). SUDs can range from moderate to severe, with addiction being the most severe.

Giving off heroin after a lengthy period of use is difficult since the body must adjust to life without it. Withdrawal symptoms normally begin 6 to 24 hours after the last dosage and persist around a week, however they can extend up to 10 days in rare cases. The first three days will be the most difficult.

- Cravings for heroin
- Restlessness and irritability
- Anxiety
- Depression and crying
- Diarrhoea
- Restless sleep and yawning
- Stomach and leg cramps
- Muscle spasms
- Vomiting and no appetite
- Goosebumps
- Hot and cold flushes
- Sweating
- Runny nose and watery eyes
- Insomnia, disturbed sleep
- Fast heartbeat are some of the most common symptoms. (Banta, 2021)

6.   METHADONE

Methadone is a medicine that has been authorized by the Food and Drug Administration (FDA) for the treatment of Opioid Use Disorder (OUD) as well as pain management. Methadone is a safe and effective medication when used as directed. Methadone assists people in achieving and maintaining recovery, as well as reclaiming active and fulfilling lives. Methadone is one part of a complete treatment strategy that involves counseling and other behavioral health therapies to provide patients a holistic approach to recovery (SAMHSA,2019).

Opioids bind to opioid receptors in the brain, causing a variety of effects ranging from pain alleviation to relaxation, pleasure, and satisfaction.

Chemical Structure of Methadone

Methadone is used as a substitute for heroin and other opioids in the treatment of opiate addiction.

Pharmacotherapy is the process of replacing a habit-forming substance with a prescription medication. Pharmacotherapy not only improves a person's wellbeing by minimizing physical withdrawal, but it also enables individuals who are addicted to heroin and other opioids to stabilize their lives and lessen the consequences associated with drug use.

Methadone relieves withdrawal symptoms in heroin or other narcotic drug addicts without creating the "high" associated with drug addiction. Methadone is a pain reliever that is also utilized in the treatment and maintenance of drug addiction. It can only be obtained from a licensed pharmacy. Methadone is a drug that is used to relieve severe pain 24 hours a day, seven days a week. This medication should not be used for pain on an as-needed basis.

Methadone relieves pain by altering the way the brain and nerve system respond to it. It takes longer for it to take action than other powerful painkillers like morphine. If you're in a lot of pain due to an injury, surgery, or long-term sickness, your doctor may prescribe methadone.

It also stops medications like codeine, heroin, hydrocodone, morphine, and oxycodone from giving you a high. It can provide a comparable sensation while also preventing withdrawal symptoms and cravings. This is referred to as replacement treatment (Kleber, 2007).

Other names

Done or 'the done'

How is it used?

Patients receiving methadone for the treatment of OUD must do so under the supervision of a medical professional. Patients may be allowed to use methadone at home between program appointments after a time of stability (based on progress and confirmed, continuous compliance with the drug dosage).

The length of time a person is treated with methadone varies. Methadone therapy should last at least 12 months, according to the National Institute on Drug Abuse publication Principles of Drug Addiction Treatment: A Research-Based Guide (Third Edition). Some patients may need to be kept on a long-term basis. To avoid withdrawal, patients must cooperate with their Medication Assisted Treatment (MAT) practitioner to gradually lower their methadone dosage .

Generally, there are two types of methadone programs:

- **Maintenance (long-term programs):** These programs might last months or years and are designed to lessen the negative consequences of drug use while also improving quality of life.
- **Short-term detoxification procedures (withdrawal):** It lasts between 5-14 days and is designed to help those who are trying to quit heroin. Methadone is a pain reliever that is given as an injection or as pills.

How effective is it?

Methadone therapy is more likely to be effective if it is part of a larger treatment plan that treats the body, mind, and environment in which heroin was used.

Treatment may involve a combination of methadone, counseling, alternative treatments, a good peer and friend support network, and a support group, for example.

Methadone maintenance may not be right for everyone, so talk to a doctor or a drug counselor to figure out what's best for you (Henry, 2003).

Advantages of methadone maintenance over **heroin use**

- Methadone maintenance keeps the person steady while they make constructive adjustments in their lives; methadone use alone is unlikely to result in an overdose.
- Health concerns, particularly those associated to injecting, such as HIV, hepatitis B and C viruses, skin infections, and vein difficulties, are decreased or prevented.
- Because methadone's effects are long-lasting, doses are only needed once a day, or even less often.
- Methadone is far less expensive than heroin.

Effects of methadone

There is no such thing as a safe amount of drug consumption. Any substance has the potential to have undesired side effects, and drugs are no exception. When using any kind of medication, it's critical to be cautious. Side effects should be regarded seriously since they might suggest a medical emergency. Patients should cease using methadone as soon as possible and notify a doctor or emergency services.

Methadone affects people differently depending on their size, weight, and health, as well as if they are acclimated to taking it and whether they are taking other medicines at the same time.

Methadone has a far longer duration of action than heroin. A single dose of morphine lasts roughly 24 hours, but a dose of heroin lasts only a few hours.

People who have had their liver function affected in the past (due to hepatitis B, hepatitis C, or long-term alcohol use) may need to be closely monitored while on methadone therapy (Henry, 2003).

Side effects

The following are the most prevalent methadone adverse effects:

- Perspiration (drink at least two litres of water each day to prevent dehydration)
- Inability to pass urine
- Nausea and vomiting, as well as a loss of appetite
- Cramping in the stomach
- Constipation
- Muscle and joint pain
- Sporadic periods
- Males with decreased sex drive
- itching and rashes
- Drowsiness, mental fogging, and perplexity

Dose-related effects

Because their dose isn't correct for them, some persons on methadone regimens can have undesirable symptoms during therapy, especially in the beginning.

If the dosage is too low, you may have the following symptoms:

- Impatience and hostility
- Lack of appetite, nausea and vomiting
- Stomach cramps and diarrhoea
- Tremors, muscular spasms, and jerks
- Back and joint pains

Overdose

The following symptoms may occur if the dosage is too high. If you or someone else experiences any of the following symptoms, call an ambulance right away (ambulance officers do not need to engage the police):

- Severe constipation with bowel blockage or inability to pass urine
- Severe allergic response with swelling of the face, lips, tongue, and neck, wheezy breathing, or tight chest
- Intense red rash with itching or hives
- Collapse

Long-term effects

Methadone in its purest form will not harm key organs, and long-term usage will not harm the body.

Withdrawal

Methadone withdrawal is less severe and takes longer than heroin withdrawal. Withdrawal symptoms are comparable to those stated under 'Dose-related consequences' under 'too low' dose in the 'too low' dose section. The majority of these side effects will appear one to three days following the last dosage, peaking around the sixth day but lasting longer.

7.   NALOXONE

Naloxone is an opioid overdose reversal drug that has been licensed by the Food and Drug Administration (FDA). It's an opioid antagonist, which means it attaches to opioid receptors and can counteract and prevent the effects of opioids like heroin, morphine, and oxycodone. Naloxone is a brief therapy that is given when a patient shows indications of an opioid overdose. Its effects do not last long. As a result, it's vital to get medical help as quickly as possible after using/receiving naloxone (SAMHSA, 2019).

Chemical Structure of Naloxone

Naloxone prescription is used to prevent or reverse the effects of opioid medications, especially in the case of drug overdoses, which are fast becoming a primary cause of mortality across the world. Naloxone has a high affinity for -opioid receptors, where it functions as an inverse agonist, leading any other medications attached to these receptors to be rapidly removed .

Opioids like morphine, hydromorphone methadone, heroin, or fentanyl, when taken in excessive doses, can cause life-threatening symptoms such respiratory depression, slowed heart rate, slurred speech, sleepiness, and constricted pupils. If left untreated, this can lead to vomiting, a lack of pulse and respiration, loss of consciousness, and death. In opioid overdose, naloxone is used to quickly reverse these signs of central nervous system depression. It's vital to remember that naloxone only works on opioid receptors in the body, therefore it won't help to reverse the effects of non-opioid drugs like methamphetamine or cocaine, or benzodiazepines like lorazepam or diazepam (SAMHSA, 2019).

Counseling Intervention

Patients will be more involved in opioid use conversations, provider satisfaction will rise, and overdoses will be reversed as a result of the counseling intervention. Improving naloxone availability is a critical component of comprehensive overdose prevention initiatives that promote safe opioid prescribing and usage.

How is it used?

Intranasal spray (into the nose), intramuscular (into the muscle), subcutaneous (under the skin), and intravenous injection are all options for administering the medicine. If a patient is getting medication-assisted treatment (MAT) or is otherwise deemed at risk for opioid overdose, a practitioner should consider prescribing naloxone. In an emergency if someone is experiencing an overdose, it can be delivered by medical experts such as paramedics, as well as family, friends, or onlookers.

It is best practice to give training to everyone who may be providing naloxone.

Effects of Naloxone

Naloxone works by temporarily blocking opioid receptors and so preventing opioid medications from acting. Because naloxone cannot be used to get high, it has no chance of being misused.

There is no indication that long-term naloxone usage can create physical damage or dependency. People who use naloxone do not build a tolerance to its effects, and no deaths from naloxone overdose have been documented.

Patients who get hives or swelling in the face, lips, or neck as a result of naloxone should seek medical attention right once. They should not drive or engage in any other potentially dangerous activities.

Naloxone usage induces opioid withdrawal symptoms. After administering/receiving naloxone, medical help should be sought as quickly as feasible.

Side effects

The majority of naloxone's adverse effects are minor. If someone is opioid-dependent and given a large dose of naloxone, they may experience symptoms of opioid withdrawal such as nausea and vomiting, sweating, shaking, anxiousness, and a quick pulse.

Even non-opioid-dependent people can have:

- An allergic response with symptoms include swelling of the face, lips, tongue, and throat, wheezy breathing, chest tightness, and a severe rash with itching
- High blood pressure
- Irregular heartbeat
- Convulsions

Naloxone and opioid overdose

People who have been revived with naloxone after an opioid overdose may feel compelled to take additional opioids, especially if they are addicted.

It is extremely risky to use opioid medicines after receiving naloxone. Naloxone has a short half-life in the body (1 to 1.5 hours), but heroin and other opioid medications have a significantly longer half-life. Sustained-release opioids like OxyContin® and MS Contin® have effects that can last up to 12 hours, thus naloxone will wear off long before the opioid has left the system. Taking additional opioids after receiving naloxone might result in a second overdose (Hedegaard, 2021).

8.   OPIUM

Opium is a highly addictive non-synthetic drug derived from the Papaver somniferum poppy plant. Many drugs, including morphine, codeine, and heroin, are derived from the opium plant. Opium is a depressive medication, meaning it slows down the transmission of information between the brain and the body (Presley et'al, 2018).

Chemical Structure of Opium

The opium poppy (Papaver somniferum L.), from which opium is extracted, is one of the first medicinal plants known to man. Although some researchers think opium usage predates Sumerian civilisation, evidence of opium production by the Sumerian people dates to 3400BCE.

Latex, a milky material found in opium poppy pods, includes a variety of compounds, including morphine and codeine. Opium is made by extracting latex from opium pods and drying it (Presley et'al, 2018).

History of Opium

For millennia, opium has been used to ease pain, and its use for surgical analgesia has been documented for generations. Opium is made from the poppy plant, Papaver somniferum. It was first planted in the Mediterranean region around 5000 B.C. and has since spread to a number of nations throughout the world. The milky fluid that leaks from the incisions in this poppy's immature seedpod has been scraped by hand and air-dried to generate opium.

The industrial poppy straw procedure of extracting alkaloids from the mature dried plant is a more recent form of harvesting for medicinal usage (concentrate of poppy straw).

It was employed as a powerful pain reliever by the ancient Greeks and Romans. The Sumerians called it "joy plant," or Hul Gil, and it was cultivated throughout Southeast Asia.

Opium was also grown by the Assyrians and Egyptians, and it migrated over the Silk Road (a network of trade routes) between Europe and China, where it was engaged in the early 1800s Opium Wars.

Opium dens were locations where opium could be purchased and sold, and they could be found all over the world, particularly in Southeast Asia, China, and Europe.

Opium dens grew established in the west, such as in San Francisco's Chinatown, then expanded east to New York in the 1800s.

For its euphoric and pain-relieving qualities, Chinese immigrants who traveled to the United States for railroad and gold rush jobs sometimes took their opium with them (WHO, 2018).

What does it look like?

Opium can be in the form of a liquid, a solid, or a powder, however most poppy straw concentrate is sold as a fine brownish powder.

Slang names

Ah-pen-yen, Aunti, Aunti Emma, Big O, Black Pill, Chandoo, Chandu, Chinese Molasses, Chinese Tobacco, Dopium, Dover's Powder, Dream Gun, Dream Stick, Dreams, Easing Powder, Fi-do-nie, Gee, God's Medicine, Gondola, Goric, Great Tobacco, Guma, Hop/hops, Joy Plant, Midnight Oil, Mira, O, O.P., Ope, Pen Yan, Pin Gon, Pox, Skee, Toxy, Toys, When-shee, Ze, and Zero.

How is opium used?

Opium can be smoked, injected intravenously, or taken as a tablet. Opium is also mixed with other substances and misused in this way. "Black," for example, is a mix of marijuana, opium, and methamphetamine, while "Buddha" is powerful marijuana laced with opium. Opium is a precursor to heroin manufacturing and may be converted into heroin.

Effects of opium

There is no such thing as a safe amount of drug consumption. Any medicine has a risk associated with it. When using any kind of medication, it's critical to be cautious.

Opium affects people differently depending on their size, weight, and health; how often they use it; if they use other drugs at the same time; how much they consume; and how strong the substance is (which varies between batches).

Opium Effect on The Mind

The euphoric effects of opium on the brain vary depending on the amount and mode of administration. When smoked, it acts rapidly because the opiate molecules enter the lungs, where they are immediately absorbed and then delivered to the brain. An opium "high" is similar to a heroin "high" in that users get a euphoric surge, followed by relaxation and pain relief.

Opium Effect on The Body

Constipation is caused by opium's inhibition of intestinal muscle action. It can also dry up the lips and nasal mucous membranes. Opium usage causes physical and psychological dependency, as well as the possibility of overdosing.

Short term effects may include:

- Exhilaration
- Relaxation
- Analgesia
- Slower, shallower breathing
- Lower heart rate
- Impaired reflexes
- Transient constipation
- Appetite loss

Overdose

You might overdose if you consume a significant amount of opium. If you or someone else has any of the following symptoms, call an ambulance immediately.

Opium overdose symptoms include:

- Very sluggish breathing
- Loss of consciousness
- Small pupils
- Seizures,
- Dizziness, weakness, death are all possible outcomes.

Overdoes that go untreated can cause brain damage and death.

Long-term effects

Regular opium usage may result in:

- Tolerance - the need to take more to have the same effect
- Irregular periods and trouble having children
- Decrease of sex desire
- Constipation
- Opium dependency

Opium and lead poisoning

- Lead contamination has been discovered in some opium.
- The source of lead in opium is unknown, however it might be due to contamination from processing equipment, purposeful adulteration of opium with lead to enhance its weight, or cultivating opium poppies in polluted soil.
- Lead poisoning can have major health consequences, including organ damage.

Mixing opium and other drugs

- Multiple depressive medications, such as **opium combined with alcohol or benzodiazepines**, can dramatically enhance the risk of overdose.
- When you combine **opium with stimulants like cocaine or speed**, your body sends opposing impulses, which can strain your heart.
- Mixing **opium and amphetamine** may also conceal their effects, increasing the danger of overdose.

Withdrawal

Giving off opium after a lengthy period of use is difficult since the body must adjust to operating without it. Opium withdrawal is comparable to withdrawal from other opioid medications.

Withdrawal symptoms often begin six to twenty-four hours after the last dosage and can continue seven to ten days. These flu-like symptoms might include:

- Restlessness and irritability
- Sleeplessness
- Depression and sobbing
- Diarrhoea
- Sweating
- Restless sleep
- Muscular cramps
- Nausea and vomiting
- Rapid heartbeat (Presley et'al, 2018).

9.   OXYCODONE

Oxycodone hydrochloride belongs to the opioid class of medicines. Opioids are any medications that operate on opioid receptors in the brain, as well as any natural or synthetic pharmaceuticals originating from or linked to the opium poppy. Opiates are a kind of opioid that is generated naturally from the opium poppy plant rather than synthetically.

Oxycodone is an opioid pain reliever. It is used to treat severe pain, such as that caused by a surgery or a traumatic accident, as well as cancer pain. Oxycodone belongs to the family of drugs known as opiate (narcotic) analgesics. It works by altering how the brain and nerve system react to pain.

It is also used to treat various forms of chronic pain after milder pain relievers such as paracetamol, ibuprofen, and aspirin have failed (Marshman et'al, 1998).

Chemical Structure of Oxycodone

Oxycodone extended-release tablets and capsules are used to treat severe pain in persons who are likely to require pain medication around the clock for a prolonged period of time and who cannot be managed with other drugs. Oxycodone extended-release tablets and capsules should not be used to relieve pain that can be treated with as-needed medicine. Oxycodone extended-release pills, capsules, and concentrated solution should only be used to treat persons who have become tolerant (accustomed to the effects of the medicine) to opioid medications after using them for at least one week.

Oxycodone is only available with a doctor's prescription. It comes in the form of slow-release pills, capsules, and a liquid that you ingest. It can also be administered through injection, however this is normally done in a hospital setting.

Oxycodone is also marketed under the trade names Oxynorm and OxyContin.

It is occasionally administered as a pill that also contains the medication naloxone (Targinact). This is used to avoid negative effects such as constipation.

However, medical professionals are becoming increasingly concerned about the hazards of utilizing these medications, particularly when they are used for an extended period of time.

Oxycodone is a Schedule 8 medication under the Pharmaceutical Benefits Scheme (PBS). This implies that while prescribing oxycodone, clinicians must follow state and territorial legislation and must inform or get clearance from the relevant health authorities (SAMHSA, 2019).

Some people take oxycodone to become drunk, which can have dangerous negative effects.

Types of oxycodone

Oxycodone is available in a variety of dosage forms, including capsules, pills, liquid, and suppositories. It is also available in a range of strengths.

Oxycodone brand names include Oxynorm®, OxyContin®, Endone®, Proladone®, and Targin®.

Other names for Hillbilly heroin include oxy, OC, and O.

How is oxycodone used?

Oxycodone is normally taken orally, although it can also be injected or used as a suppository. OxyContin® pills were modified in 2014 to prevent them from being injected by persons who abuse them. When the pills are crushed, they form a thick gel and become resistant to crushing. Even as a gel, they have controlled release qualities.

Effects of oxycodone

There is no such thing as a safe amount of drug consumption. Any medicine has some risk, and even prescriptions might cause unpleasant side effects. It is critical to exercise caution when taking any form of medication and to strictly adhere to your doctor's instructions. If you are concerned about the adverse effects of oxycodone, see your doctor.

Oxycodone affects everyone differently, however it might cause the following side effects:

- Pain alleviation
- Dizziness or faintness
- Drowsiness
- Confusion and difficulties concentrating
- Euphoria or bad mood
- Restlessness
- Stiff muscles
- Constipation
- Dry mouth
- Nausea and stomach discomfort
- Trouble urinating
- Sluggish pulse
- Excessive perspiration, flushing, and itching
- Mild allergic rash or hives (see your doctor promptly)

Injecting medications increases the risk of:

- Tetanus
- Infection
- Vein deterioration

When needles are shared, there is an increased risk of:

- Hepatitis B
- Hepatitis C and
- HIV and AIDS

Overdose

An overdose can occur if you take too much oxycodone. If you or someone else is experiencing any of these symptoms, call an ambulance immediately.

- Chest discomfort or agony
- Tiny pupils
- Reduced awareness or response
- Acute tiredness and loss of consciousness
- Lack of muscular tone or movement

Keep the medicine with you if possible so the ambulance officers know what you've taken.

Long-term effects

Regular oxycodone usage may result in:

- Dental issues
- Mood swings
- Lower sex desire and testosterone levels (males) and menstruation issues (females)
- Needing to use more to achieve the same result
- Financial, job, or social problems

Using oxycodone with other drugs

The interactions between oxycodone with other medicines can be unexpected and harmful, resulting in:

- **Oxycodone combined with alcohol** causes greater disorientation and clumsiness, as well as breathing issues.
- **Oxycodone used with some antidepressants (monoamine oxidase inhibitors - MAOIs):** delirium, convulsions, respiratory failure, coma, and death MAOIs were the first form of antidepressant to be invented, although they have now been mostly supplanted by safer and less harmful alternatives (SAMHSA, 2019).

Withdrawal

Giving off oxycodone after a lengthy period of usage is difficult since the body must adjust to life without it. It is critical to seek medical counsel, whether you have been taking it with a prescription or not.

Withdrawal symptoms fluctuate from person to person and depend on the kind of oxycodone used.

- Watery eyes
- Runny nose
- Excessive yawning
- Difficulties sleeping and extreme restlessness
- Hot and cold flushes
- Aches in muscles and joints
- Muscular spasms and tremors
- Lack of appetite, nausea and vomiting
- Elevated heart rate and blood pressure
- Uncontrolled kicking motions

Summary

Opioids are a family of chemicals produced naturally in the opium poppy plant that operate in the brain to cause a variety of effects, including pain alleviation in many cases.

Opioids can be prescribed pharmaceuticals, such as pain relievers, or they can be illegal narcotics, such as heroin.

Many prescription opioids are used to treat moderate to severe pain by blocking pain signals between the brain and the body. Opioids, in addition to relieving pain, can make some individuals feel calm, cheerful, or "high," and they can be addicted. Breathing problems, constipation, nausea, disorientation, and sleepiness are all possible adverse effects.

Opioids are all chemically linked and interact with opioid receptors on nerve cells throughout the body and brain. Opioid pain medications are typically safe when used for a short period of time and as recommended by a doctor, but because they generate euphoria in addition to pain relief, they can be misused (taken differently or in higher quantities than intended, or taken without a doctor's prescription). Regular usage, even when recommended by a doctor, can develop to dependency, and when taken inappropriately, opioid pain medications can lead to addiction, overdose events, and fatalities.

Prescription medications can help treat a variety of ailments when administered as directed by a doctor. Stimulants can aid in the treatment of attention deficit hyperactivity disorder (ADHD) and narcolepsy. Anxiety, panic, and sleep disturbances are treated using central nervous system (CNS) depressants. Opioids are used to treat chronic pain, coughing, and diarrhea. However, if these medications are abused, they can have catastrophic repercussions.

References:

1. Gowing L, Ali R, Dunlop A, Farrell M, Lintzeris N. National Guidelines for Medication-Assisted Treatmetn of Opioid Dependence. Department of Health; 2014.
2. **Banta-Green, C.J. (2021). Fentanyl data trends. Presentation to Transforming our Communities June 30, 2021.** https://youtu.be/2gyQlj-dpy8?t=685.   Slides https://adai.uw.edu/wordpress/wpcontent/uploads/youthfentanylsli des.pdf.
3. Lintzeris N, Dunlop A, Masters, D. Clinical guidelines for use of depot buprenorphine (Buvidal® and Sublocade®) in the treatment of opioid dependence. Sydney Australia: NSW Ministry of Health; 2019.
4. Cairns R, Schaffer AL, Brown JA, Pearson SA, Buckley NA. Codeine use and harms in Australia: evaluating the effects of re-scheduling. Addiction. 2019;115(3):451-9.
5. Hedegaard H, Miniño AM, Spencer MR, Warner M. Drug overdose deaths in the United States, 1999–2020. NCHS Data Brief, no 428. Hyattsville, MD: National Center for Health Statistics. 2021. DOI: https://dx.doi.org/10.15620/cdc:112340external   icon. (12/2021)
6. Substance Abuse and Mental Health Services Administration (SAMHsA) "Buprenorphine for Opiod Use Disorder" 2019 https://www.samhsa.gov/medication-assisted-treatment/medications-counseling-related-conditions/buprenorphine
7. Health Improvement Scotland "Use of long-acting injectable **buprenorphine for opioid substitution therapy"** A national position

statement SIGN publication 165 Publication date of this version: 06/04/2022 Version number: 1.0 https://www.sign.ac.uk/media/1947/buprenorphine-position-statement-sign-165.pdf

8. Van Hout MC, Rich E, Dada S, Bergin M. Codeine Is My Helper: Misuse of and Dependence on Codeine-Containing Medicines in South Africa. Qual Health Res. 2017;27(3):341-50.

9. Marshman JA, Brands B, Sproule B, Jacobs MR. Drugs & drug abuse: a reference text. 3rd ed. Marshman JA, Brands B, Sproule B, Jacobs MR, Kevin O'B F, Addiction Research Foundation of Ontario, editors. Toronto: Addiction Research Foundation; 1998.

10. Mental Health and Drug & Alcohol Office. NSW Drug and Alcohol Withdrawal Clinical Practice Guideline. NSW Department of Health; 2007, reviewed 2018.

11. National Institute for Health and Care Excellence(NIHCE). Opioid dependence: buprenorphine prolonged-release injection (Buvidal). Evidence summary [ES19]. 2019. Available from URL: https://www.nice.org.uk/advice/es19/chapter/Key-messages; https://www.sign.ac.uk/media/1947/buprenorphine-position-statement-sign-165.pdf

12. Gowing L AR, Dunlop A, Farrell M, Lintzeris N,. National Guidelines for Medication-Assisted Treatment of Opioid Dependence. Department of Health 2014 [25.08.2020].

13. Darke S, Lappin, J, & Farrell, M. The Clinician's Guide to Illicit Drugs. United Kingdom: : Silverback Publishing 2019.

14. Brands B, Sproule, B & Marshman, J, editor. Drugs & drug abuse. 3rd ed. Ontario: Addiction Research Foundation; 1998

15. Black E, Shakeshaft A, Newton N, Teesson M, Farrell M, Rodriguez D. Heroin - What you need to know. National Drug and Alcohol Research Centre: UNSW Sydney; 2014.

16. Guerin N, White V. ASSAD 2017 Statistics & Trends: Australian Secondary Students' Use of Tobacco, Alcohol, Over-the-counter

Drugs, and Illicit Substances. Centre for Behavioural Research in Cancer: Cancer Council Victoria; 2018.

17. Henry-Edwards S. Clinical guidelines and procedures for the use of methadone in the maintenance treatment of opioid dependence. 2003

18. McDonough M. Opioid treatment of opioid addiction 2013 [14.05.2021].

19. Kleber H. Pharmacologic treatments for opioid dependence: detoxification and maintenance options. Dialogues in Clinical Neuroscience. 2007;9(4).

20. Presley CC, Lindsley CW. DARK Classics in Chemical Neuroscience: opium, a historical perspective. ACS Chemical Neuroscience. 2018;9(10):2503-18.

21. World Health Organisation.Information sheet on opioid overdose Online: World Health Organisation; 2018